Guide To Cure Eye Infections

Freedom From Chronic Eye Infections

By
Dr. Elliott Charles

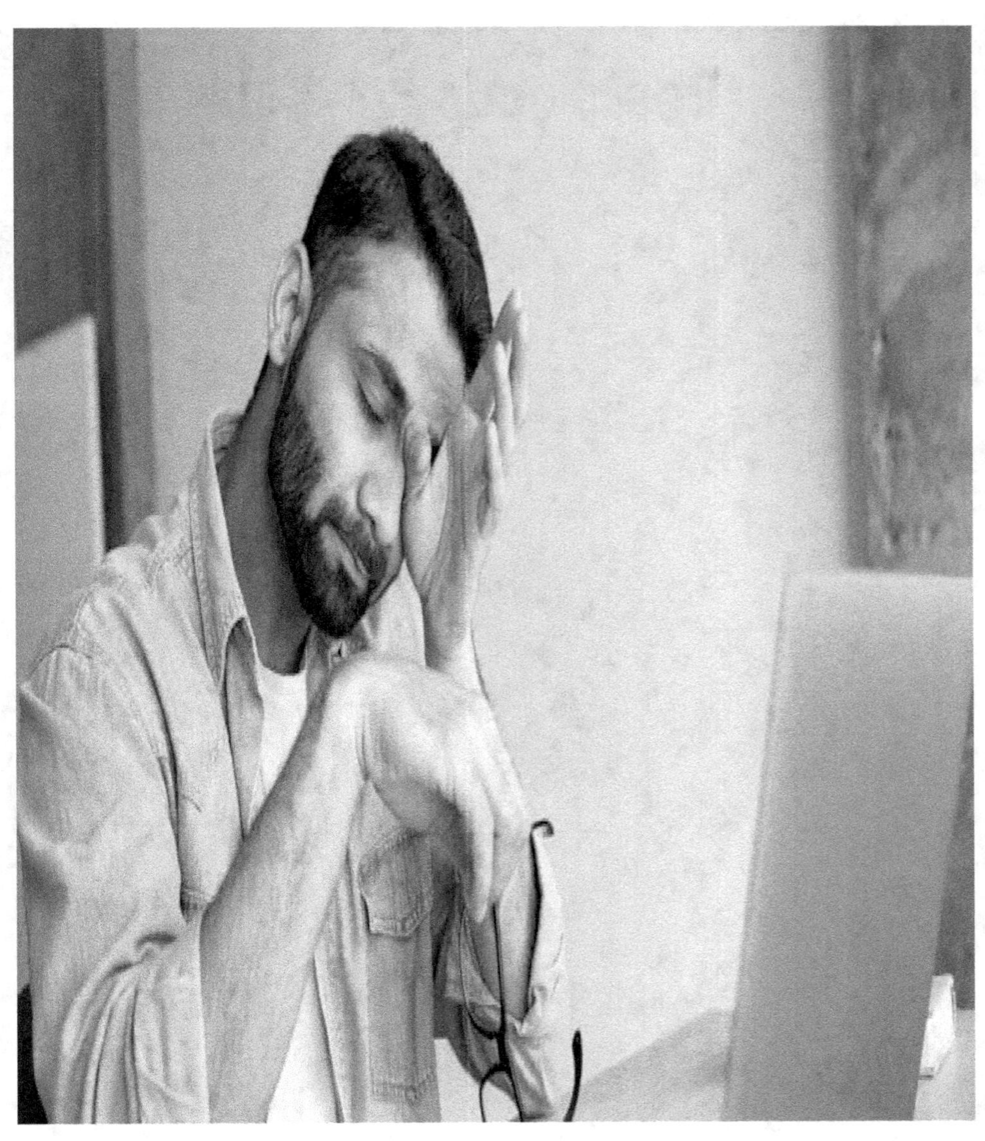

Best Foods For Your Eyes

Table Of Contents

Introduction

Refractive error is the most typical form of eye issue in the US. Examples of refractive errors that can be treated with eyeglasses, contact lenses, or, in some cases, surgery include myopia (near-sightedness), hyperopia (far-sightedness), astigmatism (distorted vision at all distances), and presbyopia (loss of ability to focus close up, inability to read phone book letters, need to hold newspaper farther away to see clearly). The National Eye Institute estimates that 150 million Americans' vision might be improved with appropriate refractive correction.

Degeneration of the macula Age-related macular degeneration (AMD), often known as macular degeneration, is a disorder that impairs crisp center vision. To perceive things and carry out daily tasks like reading and driving, one has to have a centered vision. AMD has an impact on the macula, the part of the retina in the middle that allows the eye to discern fine details. AMD comes in two flavors: dry and wet.

Wet AMD causes blood and fluid leaks because aberrant blood vessels behind the retina under the macula start to form. The bleeding, leaking, and scarring of these blood vessels result in damage and rapid central vision loss. Early symptoms of wet AMD include wavy lines appearing in straight lines.

Dry AMD is a condition that develops as people age as a result of the macula thinning, which eventually blurs central vision. The majority of AMD cases (between 70 and 90 percent) are caused by the dry form of the disease, which advances more slowly than the wet form. The damaged eye loses central vision over time as less of the macula operates. Dry AMD typically affects both eyes. One of the most prevalent early signs of dry AMD is drusen.

Under the retina, drusen are tiny white or yellow deposits. They frequently affect people over the age of 60. Small drusen are normal and do not result in vision loss. However, the risk of developing advanced dry AMD or wet AMD is increased when drusen are larger and more numerous.

An additional 7.3 million Americans with large drusen are at substantial risk of developing AMD, and it is estimated that 1.8 million Americans over the age of 40 are affected. In 2020, it is anticipated that 2.95 million people will have AMD. For people over 65, AMD is the leading cause of permanent reading and close-up or fine vision impairment.

A cataract is a clouding of the eye's lens... It is the most common cause of vision loss in the United States and the most common cause of blindness worldwide. Cataracts can be present at birth or develop at any age due to a variety of factors. Access issues like insurance coverage, treatment costs, patient choice, or a lack of awareness prevent many people from receiving the appropriate treatment for cataracts, even though the procedure is widely available.

An estimated 20.5 million Americans over the age of 40 have one or both cataracts, and 6.1 million (5.1%) have had their lenses surgically removed. By 2020, it is anticipated that the total number of people with cataracts will reach 30.1 million.

One frequent consequence associated with diabetes is diabetic retinopathy (DR). The bulk of adult blindness in the US is caused by it. Progressive damage occurs to the light-sensitive tissue at the back of the eye, which is essential for clear vision. Mild nonproliferative retinopathy (microaneurysms), moderate nonproliferative retinopathy (blockage in some retinal vessels), severe nonproliferative retinopathy (more vessels are blocked, depriving the retina of blood supply, leading to the growth of new blood vessels), and proliferative retinopathy, which is the most severe stage, are the four stages of DR. Diabetic retinopathy typically affects both eyes.

Disease management, including good control of blood sugar, blood pressure, and lipid abnormalities, reduces the risk of DR. The risk of vision loss is reduced by timely treatment and early diagnosis of DR; However, up to 50% of patients either do not have their eyes examined or are diagnosed too late to benefit from treatment.

It is the leading cause of blindness among working-age adults in the United States aged 20 to 74. Retinopathy and vision-threatening retinopathy affect an estimated 4.1 million and 899,000, respectively, Americans.

A group of diseases known as glaucoma can damage the optic nerve in the eye, which can lead to vision loss and blindness. When the normal fluid pressure inside the eyes slowly rises, glaucoma occurs. However, glaucoma can occur despite normal eye pressure, according to recent research. You can frequently safeguard your eyes from severe vision loss with prompt treatment.

There are two main types of glaucoma: open angle and closed angle. Open-angle, also known as "sneak thief of sight," is a chronic condition that progresses slowly over a long time without causing vision loss until it is very advanced. Angle-closure is a painful condition that can occur suddenly. Visual impairment can progress rapidly; However, patients seek medical attention to avoid permanent harm because of the pain and discomfort.

is sometimes referred to as "lazy eye" and is the most typical reason why kids have vision issues. The medical word for a condition where one eye's vision is compromised due to improper eye-brain communication is amblyopia. Since the brain favors the other eye, even when the eye physically seems okay, it is not being used regularly. Amblyopia can be brought on by a number of problems, one of which is strabismus, an imbalance in the position of the two eyes. less frequently, other eye disorders such cataracts, more astigmatism, nearsightedness, or farsightedness in one eye than the other.

Unless it is properly treated in early childhood, amblyopia is the most prevalent cause of permanent one-eye vision impairment in children and young and middle-aged adults. According to estimates, 2%–3% of the population suffers from amblyopia.

Strabismus refers to an unbalanced positioning of the eyes. Strabismus can cause the eyes to bend inward (esotropia) or outward (exotropia).

Strabismus is brought on by a lack of synchronization between the eyes. Hence, the eyes don't look at the same thing at the same time and look in different directions. The majority of cases of strabismus in children have no known cause. Congenital strabismus (the condition that causes the problem) is the cause of the issue in more than half of these cases. One type of amblyopia occurs when both eyes fail to focus on the same image. This results in diminished or absent depth perception, and the brain may learn to ignore the input from one eye, resulting in permanent vision loss in that eye Don't glance at the same thing and in separate directions at the same time. The majority of pediatric strabismus instances are undiagnosed. In more than half of these instances, the condition that causes the problem—congenital strabismus—is the root of the matter. When both eyes are unable to focus on the same object, one type of amblyopia develops. In addition to the brain learning to disregard the input from one eye, which could lead to permanent visual loss in that eye, this has the effect of reducing or eliminating depth awareness.

Chapter 1

Understanding The Basics Facts Of Sight

A Novel Gene-Based Eye Disorder Through genetic and clinical study, a novel macular degeneration that results in central vision loss has been identified.

The macula is a tiny portion of the retina that detects light and is essential for clear, central vision. Researchers at the National Eye Institute (NEI) have identified a new disease that affects the macula. The researchers have published their research on an unnamed new type of macular degeneration in the journal JAMA Ophthalmology. NEI is a division of the National Institutes of Health.

In macular dystrophies, abnormalities in a number of genes, including ABCA4, BEST1, PRPH2, and TIMP3, typically result in loss of central vision. For instance, Sorsby Fundus Dystrophy, a genetic eye condition directly associated to TIMP3 mutations, is commonly accompanied by adult-onset symptoms.

As a result of choroidal neovascularization, which is the development of new, atypical blood vessels beneath the retina that leak fluid and impair vision, they typically experience abrupt changes in visual acuity.

The retinal pigment epithelium (RPE), a layer of tissue that nourishes and supports the retina's light-sensing photoreceptors, secretes TIMP3, a protein that regulates blood flow in the retina. After being "cut" from RPE cells through a process known as cleavage, the mature protein contains all of the reported mutations in the TIMP3 gene.

"We were astonished that rather than in the mature protein, two patients had TIMP3 mutations in the brief signal sequence that the gene uses to "clip" the protein from the cells. According to the study's principal author, Bin Guan, Ph.D., "We demonstrated that these variations impede cleavage, resulting in the protein becoming lodged in the cell and perhaps causing toxicity to the retinal pigment epithelium." Clinical evaluations and genetic testing of family members confirmed the connection between the two new TIMP3 variants and this atypical maculopathy, as the research team followed up on these findings.

Cathy Cukras, M.D., Ph.D., a Lasker tenure-track investigator and medical retina specialist who clinically evaluated the patients, stated, "Affected individuals had scotomas or blind spots, and changes in their macules indicative of disease. However, for the time being, they have preserved central vision and no choroidal neovascularization, unlike typical Sorsby Fundus Dystrophy." The affected individuals also had changes in their macules,

To make it easier to study rare eye diseases like Sorsby Fundus Dystrophy, the NEI's Ophthalmic Genomics Laboratory collects and manages specimens as well as diagnostic data from patients who have been enrolled in numerous research projects under the NEI clinical program.

"Discovering novel disease pathways, even in known genes like TIMP3, may benefit patients who have been waiting for the correct diagnosis and will hopefully lead to new therapeutics for them," said Rob Hufnagel, M.D., Ph.D., senior author and director of NEI's Ocular Genomics Laboratory.

How might diabetes harm your eyes?

More than 4.2 million Americans over the age of 40 are either legally blind (having best-corrected visual acuity of 6/60 or worse (=20/200) in the better-seeing eye) or have low vision (having a best-corrected visual acuity of less than 6/12 (20/40) in the better-seeing eye, excluding those who were categorized as blind). Common Eye Disorders and Diseases

In the United States, age-related eye diseases like glaucoma, diabetic retinopathy, and age-related macular degeneration are the most common causes of blindness and low vision. Amblyopia and strabismus are two other common eye conditions.

Refractive Mistakes

In the United States, the most common type of eye problem is a refractive error. Myopia (near-sightedness), hyperopia (farsightedness), astigmatism (distorted vision at all distances), and presbyopia (loss of ability to focus close up, inability to read phone book letters, need to hold newspaper farther away to see clearly) are examples of refractive errors that can be corrected with eyeglasses, contact lenses, or, in some cases, surgery. According to the National Eye Institute, 150 million Americans could see better with proper refractive correction.

**What warning indications are there that you may
have refractive errors?**

Presbyopia affects the majority of adults over the
age of 35. Age-Related Macular Degeneration
Macular degeneration, also known as age-related
macular degeneration (AMD), is an eye disorder that
is associated with aging and causes damage to sharp
and central vision. It is necessary to have a central
vision in order to clearly see things and perform
everyday activities like reading and driving. The
macula, the central portion of the retina that enables
the eye to see fine details, are affected by AMD.
There are two types of AMD: moist and dry.

Under the macula, abnormal blood vessels behind
the retina begin to grow, resulting in blood and fluid
leakage in wet AMD. Damage and rapid central
vision loss are caused by these blood vessels'
bleeding, leaking, and scarring. The appearance of
wavy lines in straight lines is an early sign of wet
AMD.

As part of the aging process, dry AMD occurs when
the macula gradually thins, gradually blurring
central vision. The dry form of AMD, which
progresses more slowly than the wet form, is more
prevalent and accounts for 70–90 percent of cases.
As less of the macula functions over time, the

affected eye gradually loses its central vision. In most cases, dry AMD affects both eyes. Drusen is one of the most common early symptoms of dry AMD.

Under the retina, drusen are tiny white or yellow deposits. They frequently affect people over the age of 60. Small drusen are normal and do not result in vision loss. However, the risk of developing advanced dry AMD or wet AMD is increased when drusen are larger and more numerous.

An additional 7.3 million Americans with large drusen are at substantial risk of developing AMD, and it is estimated that 1.8 million Americans over the age of 40 are affected. In 2020, it is anticipated that 2.95 million people will have AMD. For people over 65, AMD is the leading cause of permanent reading and close-up or fine vision impairment.

What are the AMD risk factors?
Pregnancy being Latino or African American Cigarette Cataract Cataracts are the primary cause of vision loss in the US and the primary cause of blindness worldwide. Diabetes type 1 or type 2 poor management of blood sugar high cholesterol and blood pressure.

Cataracts can be present at birth or develop at any age due to a variety of factors. Access issues like insurance coverage, treatment costs, patient choice, or a lack of awareness prevent many people from receiving the appropriate treatment for cataracts, despite the fact that the procedure is widely available.

An estimated 20.5 million Americans over the age of 40 have one or both cataracts, and 6.1 million (5.1%) have had their lenses surgically removed. By 2020, it is anticipated that the total number of people with cataracts will reach 30.1 million.

What are the cataract risk factors?
diabetic eye disease One typical consequence of diabetes is diabetic retinopathy (DR). Retinopathy accounts for the majority of adult blindness in the United States. The light-sensitive tissue at the back of the eye, which is necessary for good vision, is progressively damaged in this condition. There are four stages of DR: mild nonproliferative retinopathy (microaneurysms), moderate nonproliferative retinopathy (blockage in some retinal vessels), severe nonproliferative retinopathy (more vessels are blocked, depriving the retina of blood supply, leading to the growth of new blood vessels), and

proliferative retinopathy, which is the most severe stage. Both eyes are typically impacted by diabetic retinopathy.

Disease management, including good control of blood sugar, blood pressure, and lipid abnormalities, reduces the risk of DR. The risk of vision loss is reduced by timely treatment and early diagnosis of DR; However, up to 50% of patients either do not have their eyes examined

are identified when it is too late to receive therapy.

It is the leading cause of blindness among working-age adults in the United States aged 20 to 74. Retinopathy affects an estimated 4.1 million Americans, while vision-threatening retinopathy affects 899,000.

A group of diseases known as glaucoma can damage the optic nerve in the eye, which can lead to vision loss and blindness. Glaucoma develops as the normally-occurring fluid pressure inside the eyes gradually increases. Recent studies have found that glaucoma can still develop in the presence of normal eye pressure. Often, quick treatment can protect your eyes from serious vision loss.

Open-angle and closed-angle glaucoma are the two primary varieties. Open-angle, also known as "sneak thief of sight," is a chronic condition that progresses slowly over a long period of time without causing vision loss until it is very advanced. Angle-closure is a painful condition that can occur suddenly. Visual impairment can progress rapidly; However, patients seek medical attention in order to avoid permanent harm because of the pain and discomfort.

What are the risk factors for glaucoma?
 Glaucoma can affect anyone, but some people are more likely to get it.
Amblyopia, also known as "lazy eye," is the most common cause of vision impairment in children and affects everyone over the age of 60, especially Mexican Americans and African Americans over 40. Amblyopia is the medical term for a condition in which the eye and brain are not working together properly, resulting in decreased vision in one eye. The eye itself appears normal, but the brain is favoring the other eye, so it is not being used normally. strabismus, which is an imbalance in the position of the two eyes, is one of the conditions that can cause amblyopia. more astigmatism, nearsightedness, or farsightedness in one eye than in the other, and rarely other eye conditions like cataracts.

Amblyopia

Amblyopia is the most common cause of permanent one-eye vision impairment in children and young and middle-aged adults unless it is successfully treated in early childhood. Amblyopia affects about 2%–3% of the population, according to estimates.

Chapter 2

Early warning signs And Causes Of Eye Problem

The majority of people will experience eye issues at some point in their lives. Some are minor and can be treated at home or will go away on their own. Some people require specialized care.

There are things you can do to get your eye health back on track, whether your vision isn't as good as it used to be or never was.

Check to see if any of these common issues ring a bell. If your symptoms are severe or do not improve within a few days, always consult a doctor.

Eyestrain

Eye strain is well-known to anyone who spends long periods of time reading, working at a computer, or driving. It occurs when you use your eyes too much. Just like any other part of your body, they get tired and need to rest. If your eyes feel strained, give them some time off. Check with your doctor to make sure there isn't another issue if they still feel tired after a few days.

eye color

Your eyes appear red. Why?

When infected or irritated, blood vessels that cover their surface expand. That makes your eyes appear red.

It can be caused by eye strain, late nights, insufficient sleep, or allergies. Consult your doctor if the problem is caused by an injury.

Red eyes could be a sign of conjunctivitis (pinkeye), which is another eye infection, or sun damage from not wearing shades for too long. Consult your doctor if rest and eye drops purchased over the counter do not help.

Night Blindness Is it difficult to see at night, particularly when driving?

Is it difficult to navigate dark environments like movie theaters?

That makes me think of night blindness. It is a symptom rather than a standalone issue. Night blindness is a condition that can be corrected by doctors and is caused by nearsightedness, cataracts, keratinous, and deficiencies in vitamin A.

This issue can occur in some people from birth or as a result of a retinal degenerative disease that usually cannot be treated. If you have it, you will need to be even more careful in low-light settings.

Slow Eye

When one eye does not grow normally, it is known as amblyopia or lazy eye. That eye's vision is worse, and it tends to "lazily" move around while the other eye stays put. Rarely affecting both eyes, it affects adults, children, and infants. Children and infants require immediate medical attention.

If a lazy eye is discovered and treated in early childhood, it can prevent vision problems that last a lifetime. The use of a patch or other methods to get a child to use the lazy eye, as well as corrective glasses or contact lenses, are all options for treatment.

Nystagmus as well as crossed eyes (strabismus)
Cross Eyes (Strabismus) and Nystagmus If you look at something with your eyes not aligned, you may have strabismus. It may also be referred to as walleye or crossed eyes.

This issue cannot be resolved by itself. With the help of an eye doctor, you might be able to participate in vision therapy to strengthen the weak eye muscles. You might have to see an ophthalmologist or eye surgeon to have it fixed surgically. It will need to be fixed by an ophthalmologist, also known as an eye specialist.

The eye moves or "jiggles" constantly on its own in nystagmus.

There are numerous treatments, such as vision therapy to strengthen your eyes. Surgery is another choice. To determine which treatment might be most effective for you, your doctor will examine your eyes.

Color Blindness

You may be colorblind if you can't see or tell the difference between certain colors (usually red and green). It occurs when your eye's color cells, also known as cone cells, are missing or do not function properly.

You can only see in gray tones at its worst, but this is uncommon. The majority of people who have it are born with it, but some drugs and diseases can cause it later in life. You can find out what's to blame from your doctor. Men are much more likely than women to be born with it.

Your eye doctor can identify it with a simple test. If you were born with it, there is no cure, but special contacts and glasses can help some people tell different colors apart.

The term "uveitis" refers to a group of conditions that result in inflammation of the uvea. The majority of the eye's blood vessels are located in that middle layer.

Eye tissue can be destroyed and even lost as a result of these diseases. People of all ages can access it. It's possible for symptoms to go away quickly or for a long time.

Uveitis

Uveitis may be more common in people with immune system conditions like AIDS, rheumatoid arthritis, or ulcerative colitis. Some of the signs could be:

Symptoms such as blurred vision, eye pain, redness, and light sensitivity should be reported to your doctor if they persist beyond a few days. Depending on the type of uveitis you have, different treatments are available.

Presbyopia

Presbyopia occurs when, despite having good distance vision, you lose the ability to clearly see close objects and small print.

To make it easier to read, you may need to hold a book or other reading material further away from your eyes after around 40. Similar to your arms being too short.

Restoring good reading vision can be accomplished with the help of reading glasses, contact lenses, and other procedures.

Floaters

Floaters are minuscule specks or spots that float across your field of vision. The majority of people notice them outdoors in bright sunlight or in well-lit rooms.

Floaters are typically normal, but they may occasionally indicate a more serious eye condition, such as retinal detachment. The back of your eye's retina separates from the layer below it at that point. Along with the floaters, you might also see light flashes or a dark shadow cross the edge of your vision when this happens.

Dry Eyes

When your eyes can't make enough good-quality tears, you get dry eyes. You might feel as though something is burning in your eye. Extreme dryness can occasionally result in partial vision loss in severe cases. Among the treatments are:
Use a home humidifier Special eye drops that mimic real tears and Plugs in your tear ducts to reduce

drainage Lipiflow, a procedure that treats dry eyes with heat and pressure, Testosterone eyelid cream Dietary supplements containing fish oil and omega-3 To help you make more tears, your doctor might give you drops like cyclosporine (Cequa, Restasis), lifitegrast (Xiidra), or Tyrvaya nose spray.

Excess Tearing

Excessive crying is unrelated to your emotions. You might be sensitive to changes in temperature, wind, or light. Try to shield your eyes or wear sunglasses to protect them (go with wraparound frames because they block more wind than other types).

Tearing could also be a sign of something more serious, like an infection in the eye or a clogged tear duct.
Your eye doctor is able to treat or remedy both of these issues.

Cataracts

A healthy lens is as transparent as a camera's. Cloudy spots called cataracts develop in the eye. It carries light to your retina, which is part of your eye that processes images at the back. Light can't pass through as easily when you have a cataract. The outcome: You may notice glare or a halo around lights at night because you can't see as well.

Usually, cataracts form slowly. They do not result in eye irritation, redness, or pain.

Some remain small and do not impair your vision. Surgery almost always restores vision if they progress and affect it.

Glaucoma

A tire is like your eye: It has normal and safe pressure in certain places. However, excessive levels can harm your optic nerve. A group of diseases that cause glaucoma is called glaucoma.

Primary open-angle glaucoma is a common type. The majority of people who have it do not experience pain or early symptoms. Therefore, it is essential to maintain regular eye examinations.

Despite its rarity, glaucoma can be brought on by:

Retinal Disorders

Disorders of the retina are a thin lining on the back of your eye that is made up of cells that collect images and send them to your brain. Inflammatory

disorders of the eye Retinal Disorders Disorders of the retina can damage the cells in the retina and prevent this transfer. There are various varieties:
The macula, a small portion of the retina, is destroyed in age-related macular degeneration.
Diabetes-related damage to the blood vessels in your retina is known as diabetic retinopathy.
When the retina separates from the layer below it, this condition is known as retinal detachment.
Getting these conditions treated and diagnosed early is critical.

Conjunctivitis (Pinkeye) (Pinkeye)
The tissue that lines the inside of your eyelids and covers your sclera gets inflamed when you have this illness. Possible adverse effects include redness, burning, stinging, tearing, discharge, or the impression that something is in your eye.
People of all ages can access it. Allergies, infection, and exposure to irritants and toxins are all potential causes.

Wash your hands often to lower your risk of catching it.
Eye Illnesses

Diseases of the cornea are your eyes clear, dome-shaped "window." Focusing on the light that comes in is helpful. It can be damaged by disease, infection, injury, and exposure to toxins. Some warnings are:

Eyes that are red and watery have pain, blurry vision, or a halo effect. The main treatments are as follows:

A new prescription for eyeglasses or contacts Medicated eye drops Surgery Eyelid issues Your eyelids are very important to you. They limit the amount of light that can enter your eye, spread tears across its surface, and protect it.

Eyelid issues frequently manifest as sensitivity to light, pain, itching, and tearing. Additionally, you may have inflamed outer edges near your eyelashes or blinking spasms.

Proper cleaning, medication, or surgery are all options for treatment.

Changes in vision As you get older, it's possible that you won't be able to see as well as you used to. That is typical. Most likely, you'll need contacts or glasses. To improve your vision, you may decide to undergo surgery (LASIK). If you already wear glasses, your prescription might need to be stronger.

As you get older, you also get other, more serious diseases. Vision problems can be caused by eye diseases like macular degeneration, glaucoma, and cataracts. Keep up with your eye exams because these disorders have very different symptoms.

Some changes in vision can be dangerous and necessitate immediate medical attention. See a doctor right away if you experience a sudden loss of vision or if everything appears blurry, even if it is only temporary.

They are effective for many individuals, but you must maintain them. Before you use your hands, wash them. Care instructions that come with your prescription should be followed. And adhere to these guidelines:

Never put them in your mouth to get them wet. That could raise the risk of infection.

Make sure the lenses fit correctly to avoid scratching your eyes.

Make sure the eye drops you use are safe for contact lenses.

Never make saline solutions from scratch. Even though some lenses have been approved by the FDA to be worn while sleeping, doing so increases the likelihood of a serious infection.

Consult your eye doctor if you do everything right but still have issues with your contacts. You might need glasses because you have dry eyes, allergies, or both. You can decide what is best for you once you understand the issue.

Eye Issues' Symptoms And Indicators

1.Double Vision Double vision is a problem that should be taken seriously right away, regardless of whether it occurs on a regular basis or at random. A person experiencing it will see two images stacked on top of one another or next to each other. It can immediately impede reading, maintaining equilibrium, and performing daily tasks. It is monocular when it only affects one eye, but binocular when it affects both. It can be brought on by a number of underlying conditions, including diseases that weaken the eye muscles and damage to nerves and muscles. It could also occur as a result of drinking or using drugs. It is a symptom that must be evaluated and treated right away if it persists without alcohol or drugs.

2. Eye Pain is a common sign. Eye pains that throb, stab, or shoot may be what identify it. Trauma, irritation from a foreign object (something is stuck in your eye), infection, or another serious underlying condition can all cause it.

The pain in your eye is not normal. It may be an acute issue that does not indicate an underlying condition if it occurs rarely when combined with other symptoms like a headache. However, if you experience it frequently, you should see an eye doctor because it could indicate anything from nerve damage or inflammation.

3. Scratchy Pain On The Eye Surface A foreign object, like a piece of sand or a small hair, frequently causes scratching pain on the eye's surface. It could also be a sign of dry eyes, in which your eyelids irritate the cornea's surface every time you blink and your eyes are not adequately lubricated.

When the foreign object leaves the eye, this may go away, but if it keeps happening, it could be a sign of a problem that needs treatment. Therefore, do not disregard it! Your physician is able to identify the issue and treat the underlying condition to alleviate it.

4. Floaters or Spots Everybody at some point sees floaters or spots, which typically appear when looking at bright lights. However, for some individuals, it is more severe, frequent, and persistent. Age is frequently the cause of floating objects, which are small objects that move around in your field of vision. The vitreous fluid in your eyes becomes more fluid as you get older and your eyes slowly deteriorate. If you experience an excessive number, however, it could be a sign of an underlying condition like inflammation in the back of the eye, a torn retina, or bleeding. The minute fibers in that fluid begin to clump together over time, creating shadows on the retina. If you notice more floaters than usual, start seeing flashes of light, or start seeing darkness or dark spots in your vision, you should see a doctor.

5. Impaired peripheral vision Your ability to see out of the corner of your eye or in areas where you aren't focusing is called peripheral vision. It's possible that you have optic nerve damage from glaucoma if you find that you can't see what's around you, either on one side or both.
This issue can also be caused by eye occlusions, which prevent the regular flow of blood to the optic

nerve and other parts of the eye. If you have trouble seeing in the distance, you should get your eyes checked right away.

6. Narrowed Field Of Vision A person with a narrowed field of vision may only be able to see what is directly in front of them, which is similar to having impaired peripheral vision. It might start out as a problem with peripheral vision and progress to tunnel vision, which makes it feel like you're looking through a hole.

See a doctor right away if you start to notice that your field of vision is getting smaller.It can also be a sign of glaucoma.
7. Stomas, or blind spots, can appear anywhere in your vision. They might show up as a dark spot in the middle of your vision or on the edges of it. It could also appear as a moving, flickering light in the middle of your eye that moves around. Migraines may result from these brief activities, or they may last a lifetime.

A stroke, tumor, trauma, glaucoma, multiple sclerosis, or exposure to toxic chemicals are all potential causes of these blind spots.

8. Swelling Around the eye, however, swelling can be brought on by a wide range of other issues that your eye doctor can accurately diagnose. Swelling in the eye can present symptoms similar to those we discussed earlier. Allergies, fluid retention, or serious eye infections that can cause permanent damage if untreated can cause swelling.

Eyelid swelling can also be a sign of serious health issues like Graves' disease, ocular herpes, or orbital cellulitis, all of which have the potential to permanently impair vision.

Eye Health Risk Factors

Factors that increase eye health risk When should I have my eyes examined?

Have your eyes examined whenever you or a loved one experience vision issues.

Some adults and children may be more likely to develop eye problems because of their age, certain medical conditions, or family history. A comprehensive baseline exam and guidance on how frequently to have follow-up exams should be obtained from an ophthalmologist or optometrist for adults (and children) at risk for vision issues.

These are risk factors for eye health:

Age-related diseases including glaucoma and cataracts start to manifest more commonly. According to Safe Eyes USA, every adult over the age of 40 should undergo a thorough baseline eye checkup. As people age, glaucoma and cataracts grow increasingly prevalent, and most people begin to have near vision issues (presbyopia).

Adults with diabetes should have their eyes checked annually, and more frequently if diabetes-related abnormalities are discovered. Whether or not individuals experience any eye symptoms, this is true.

Adult blindness and vision loss are primarily brought on by diabetes and its effects on the eye. Problems can be detected before they get worse by performing the recommended tests. Vision loss can be avoided with early treatment, such as better blood sugar control, laser treatment, and injections.

Hypertension is high blood pressure.
If you have high blood pressure, you should get your eyes checked. The blood vessels in the retina, which is the back of the eye, can change if you have high blood pressure. Using eye exams, you can see and track these changes. Additionally, hypertension is a

risk factor for the onset or progression of eye diseases like diabetic retinopathy, glaucoma, and macular degeneration.

An eye disease in the family history

Your risk of acquiring an eye condition may be higher than usual if your family has a history of glaucoma, macular degeneration, cataracts at a young age, or other eye conditions. For instance, if glaucoma runs in a person's family, they are four to nine times more likely to get the condition. Get an eye test and learn about your family's history of eye problems if you believe you may be at risk.

Some Risks For Children

As part of good well-child care, pediatricians and family doctors should regularly screen children's eyes. School-based vision screenings should be given to older children. The vast majority of children do not require comprehensive examinations, saving their families time and money as well as preventing the children from having to take part in tests that are not necessary.

If a child fails a routine screening or exhibits risk factors for potential eye conditions, they should be referred to an eye doctor for a comprehensive exam. Children's eye health risk factors include:

Why is prompt diagnosis crucial?
One of the most crucial justifications for getting an eye checkup is to maintain the health of your eyes. When people consider obtaining an eye exam, many of them picture getting a new prescription for glasses or contacts. There is much more to it than just having a properly calibrated prescription for good vision. Preventing eye infections or limiting damage to the eyes from undiagnosed eye diseases is one of the primary justifications for getting an eye exam.

Numerous eye conditions and issues are silent. This indicates that the person experiencing the issue is unable to identify it early on. Many people believe that if something is wrong with their eyes, they will know. Even though this is sometimes the case, routine eye exams can reveal conditions like glaucoma, macular degeneration, diabetic retinopathy, cataracts, and retinal detachments. Preventing sight loss can be accomplished with prompt treatment.

Chapter 3

Prevention And Treatment Of Eye Infections

What common eye conditions can I prevent?

Most people consider sight to be the most practical sense. It can help you perceive and manage your surroundings more effectively. As a result, maintaining your eyes' functionality requires proper care.

Most people occasionally experience vision problems, which often worsen as they age. The majority of these problems are minor and transient. Yet, there are several major eye conditions that can cause the eyes significant harm, including the permanent loss of eyesight.

Fortunately, most eye problems, even the most serious ones, can be avoided. Some common eye problems that can be prevented are listed here.

How to Prevent It

In most cases, increased tear evaporation can be avoided. Exposure to wind, smoke, or dry air is the common factor that contributes to an increase in tear evaporation. On dry, windy days, wearing sunglasses to protect your eyes can help prevent dry eyes. If you work outdoors in dry, windy, or smokey conditions, you can also wear goggles.

Dry eyes can also result from not blinking enough. When you focus on reading, driving, or working on a computer for an extended period of time, this can happen. Take brief breaks from your work to rest your eyes to prevent this.

Additionally, eye drops are useful in preventing dry eyes. Vitamin A and cyclosporine drops, according to research, can significantly alleviate dry eye symptoms. Preservative-free artificial tear eye drops were found to be less effective than these kinds of drops.

Although dry eye is not a dangerous condition in and of itself, it can lead to serious eye conditions like infections and damage.

Treatments for Refractive Errors
Surgical Treatments

LASIK – This highly effective laser eye surgery procedure uses state-of-the-art, computer-guided lasers to create a flap in the top layer of the cornea and to reshape the cornea. You can avoid developing dry eyes if you are exposed to situations that can cause them by gently cleaning your eyelids with a towel and warm water. PRK is a minimally invasive method of reshaping the cornea that is comparable to LASIK. In contrast to LASIK, the cornea's top layer is gently removed and left to regenerate on its own for two to four days.

Vision ICL: An implantable collier lens is inserted between the iris and natural lens, rather than reshaping the cornea.
Non-surgical treatments for

Presbyopia cures in OKC Surgical remedies

Surgery for presbyopia in OKC When an artificial intraocular lens (IOL) is utilized to replace the natural lens in the eye, the procedure is known as a "custom lens replacement."
During this customized LASIK surgery, one eye's distance vision and the other eye's near vision are both corrected.

How to treat cataracts

Laser cataract surgery removes the clouded lens and replaces it with a clear intraocular lens using the same computer-guided technology as LASIK (IOL)

Keratinous treatments Surgical procedures

Treatments for Keratinous Surgical treatments Corneal Collagen Cross-Linking (CXL) – Riboflavin eye drops are combined with ultraviolet light to induce the crosslinking of corneal collagen and strengthen the cornea. Monovision contact lenses Multifocal contact lenses Reading glasses

Intakes is a novel alternative to corneal transplant surgery that reshapes and flattens the cornea without removing any corneal tissue. Thin inserts are placed around the cornea's outer edge.

An intraplate femtosecond laser is used in Intraplate-enabled keratopathy (IEK) to replace a diseased or damaged cornea with healthy tissue from a donor cornea.

Treatments that are not surgical include soft contact lenses (for mild to moderate keratinous) and rigid gas permeable (RGP) lenses for age-related macular degeneration.

Age-related macular degeneration treatments

Although AMD cannot be cured, there are treatments that can delay or stop visual loss.

Surgical procedures Anti-VEGF drug injections - Anti-VEGF drug injections assist lower the number of aberrant blood vessels in the retina and decrease the leakage of vessels.

A unique laser therapy called photodynamic laser therapy (PDT) promotes the disintegration of the aberrant blood vessels in the retina.

procedures that don't involve surgery big print materials and magnifiers are examples of vision aids.

vitamins and dietary supplements such as beta-carotene, zinc, copper, vitamin C, and vitamin E anti-angiogenic drugs that help to stop the development of new or leaky blood vessels.

Treatments for Diabetic Retinopathy
Surgical treatments
Scatter laser surgery (photocoagulation) is one surgical treatment for diabetic retinopathy. In this in-office procedure, lasers are used to shrink the blood vessels in the eye by burning the areas where the retina has separated from the macula.
Vitrectomy: This procedure removes the vitreous gel that covers the eye and makes it possible to make a number of repairs to the retina and macula.
Injecting anti-VEGF medications can slow the leaking of vessels and reduce the number of abnormal blood vessels in the retina.
Steroid injections are used to treat inflammation in the eye with corticosteroids.

Treatments for Diabetic Retinopathy
Surgical treatments
Trabeculoplasty is a straightforward surgical treatment for open-angle glaucoma that directs

lasers at the drainage tissue of the eye to encourage fluid drainage.

A trabeculectomy is a surgical procedure for open-angle glaucoma in which extra fluid is removed from the eye through a small opening made in the eye's top under the eyelid.

A group of treatments for mild cases of glaucoma known as MIGS (minimally invasive glaucoma surgery) makes use of microscopic instruments and tiny incisions.

Several types of glaucoma can be treated with glaucoma implant surgery, which involves inserting tiny tubes into the eye to drain fluid and relieve pressure.

Non-invasive treatments

Prescription eye drops: Depending on the type of eye drop used, the eye may be able to drain fluid more effectively or create less of it.

Therapies for Retinal Tears & Detachments

Therapies for Tears and Retinal Detachment In order to maintain safe and healthy eyesight, retinal detachment is a medical emergency that needs to be attended to immediately. A retinal detachment or tear almost always requires surgical treatment.

Laser Surgery (photocoagulation): When a retinal tear has not progressed to a detachment, this procedure uses lasers to burn around the tear and "weld" it back to the underlying tissue.

Another treatment for retinal tears, freezing (cryopexy) involves applying a freezing probe to the eye's outer surface to create scar tissue that binds the retina to the eye wall.

Pneumatic retinopexy is a treatment for retinal detachments that involves injecting a gas bubble into the eye to push the retina back into place while a laser or cryopexy seals it up.

Scleral buckling:

 A scleral buckle is a small, flexible band that is positioned around the white part of the eye (the sclera). It helps the retina reattach by pushing the sides of the eye inward.

Vitrectomy: This procedure removes the vitreous gel that lines the eye and makes it possible for the doctor to use cryopexy, pneumatic retinopexy, or laser treatment to fix the retina.

Strabismus treatments

The length or position of the muscles that control eye movement can be changed surgically to straighten the eyes.

Treatments that don't require surgery Eye exercises: By teaching the brain and eyes to work together more effectively, a structured program of visual activities can help improve eye coordination and focus.

Contact lenses or eyeglasses: Corrective lenses improve visual focus and reorient the line of vision, allowing the eyes to straighten.

Prism lenses are specialized lenses that change how images reach the eye by being thicker on one end.

Eye patches: By forcing the weaker eye to focus correctly, covering the normal-functioning or dominant eye can strengthen the weaker eye.

Drops for the eyes: Medicated drops that blur the vision in the stronger eye make it harder for the weaker eye to focus properly.

Injections: Medication injected into the eye can temporarily paralyze or weaken an overactive eye muscle.

Treatments for Amblyopia

Eye drops for amblyopia treatment: Medicated drops that make the stronger eye blur make the weaker eye compensate and focus properly.

Eye patch: If the normal eye is covered, the brain may be forced to use the weaker eye to see.

Chapter 4

Tried And Tested Natural And Home Remedies For Eye Problem

Certain home cures might be beneficial, depending on the severity of the ailment. You likely have an eye infection if your eyes are always dry and itching. Eye infections can result in serious health issues, as well as discomfort and anguish, if left untreated. Fortunately, you can use home remedies for eye infections in addition to traditional medicine to get rid of them. Continue reading to learn more!

How Can Eye Infections Happen?
Eye infections are frequently indicated by redness and itching in the eyes.
Certain areas of your eyes could be impacted:
Eye infections are frequently brought on by the eyelids, cornea, and conjunctiva (the region that covers the eye's inner and outer layers).
Blepharitis is an irritated and crusty eyelid.
When the tear ducts do not produce enough lubricant, dry eyes develop, causing discomfort and redness of the eyes.
The cornea is inflamed in keratitis.
Pink eye, which is also known as conjunctivitis, is caused by irritation or inflammation of the conjunctiva. It causes redness, itching, and tears to come out of the eyes.
Style is a red, painful lump that looks like a boil or pimple and is located close to the edge of the eyelid.
Any or both of your eyes can be affected by an eye infection. According to Dr. Michael J. Shumski,

MD, MSE, one of the best cataract and refractive surgeons, "contact lens-related infections are one of the most common infections that can cause permanent vision damage and blindness." Many different kinds of bacteria can be spread by wearing contact lenses. In otherwise healthy young adults, these are some of the most prevalent infections that can cause blindness and vision loss.

Home remedies can alleviate symptoms and assist in infection management, despite the importance of medication. Make sure you talk to your doctor about these treatments.

Eye Infection Home Remedies

1 Colostrum, or milk from the mother, can cause eye infections in newborns. Conjunctivitis, a common neonatal eye infection, can be effectively treated with breast milk. Antibodies that can help fight infections and alleviate conjunctivitis in newborn babies are abundant in the colostrum.

You will require a few drops of breast milk. With a dropper, pour a few drops of colostrum into the infant's eyes.

 In five minutes, wash your eyes.

How Often Should You Perform This? Perform this twice daily.

The initial milk that the mammary glands generate after childbirth is called colostrum, according to StyleCraze trivia. The best foods to increase breast milk supply Pumped colostrum can be stored in the freezer for six to twelve months and used whenever necessary due to its superior effectiveness against eye infections over mature milk (1).

2. Essential Oils The essential oils of rosemary, peppermint, and tea tree are antimicrobial. As a result, they might aid in the fight against and prevention of bacterial infections.

You'll need 1 liter of hot water, a few drops of rosemary or tea tree oil, a towel, and three to four drops of essential oil. Heat the water in a large bowl. Bend over the bowl while covering yourself with a towel.

Give your skin five to six minutes to soak up the steam.

How Often Should You Perform This? Perform this twice daily.

Caution: Do not apply diluted or undiluted essential oils to the eyes because they may irritate and cause burning.

3. Green Tea Bags The extract of green tea contains a lot of bioactive compounds with anti-inflammatory properties (3). Green tea bags may reduce swelling and soothe your eyes, but there is no scientific evidence that they can treat eye infections. As a result, be cautious.

You will need two bags of green tea. What you need to do is take two bags of used green tea.

Place them on your eyes for 15 to 20 minutes and refrigerate them.

Wash your eyes and take them out.

How Often Should You Perform This? To lessen the pain and swelling, perform this two times per day.

Stylecraze advises throwing out used teabags right away to prevent the infection from spreading to other eyes or people.

4. Honey Eye infections like blepharitis, keratitis and keratoconjunctivitis have all been treated with honey (4). Honey may alleviate eye infections due to its anti-inflammatory and antimicrobial properties.

A sterilized dropper, two teaspoons of honey, and one cup of water are all you'll need. All you have to do is boil one cup of water and add a few drops of honey to it.

Give it a good stir and let it cool down.

Put a drop in each eye with a clean dropper.

After five minutes, rinse with water.

How Often Should You Perform This?

Display this at least twice per day.

5. Turmeric The most important bioactive ingredient in turmeric is curcumin. The symptoms of eye infections may be alleviated by its anti-inflammatory and antimicrobial properties (5). The initial studies have shown promising results, despite the fact that additional randomized clinical trials are required to establish its therapeutic properties. As a result, turmeric may be an effective home remedy for eye infections.

You will need one teaspoon of turmeric powder and one cup of warm water. What to do: Boil one cup of water and add one teaspoon of turmeric.

Give it some time to cool down.

Put a clean washcloth in this solution and soak it.

Wash your eyes afterward and apply this as a warm compress.

6. How Often Should You Perform It? Perform this at least once per day.

Related: How to Use Turmeric, Its 18 Health Benefits, and Its Side Effects Lemon Juice Eye infections can sometimes recur as a result of allergic reactions to certain substances or a change in the weather. Lemon juice can aid in the treatment of eye infections and their symptoms due to its antioxidant and anti-inflammatory properties (6). But because there isn't enough research to support this, you should talk to your doctor about this remedy.

You will need one glass of warm water and one-half of a ripe lemon. What to do: Extract the lemon juice.

Mix well this into a glass of warm water.

Take this all in.

How Often Should You Drink This Juice? Consume this juice at least once per day.

7. Certain kinds of eye infections can be treated with saline water (7). Saline's antiseptic properties may be to blame, according to some. Nevertheless, there is no study to back this up.

statement. Some claim that saline water can aid in the treatment of eye infections due to its similarity to teardrops.

You'll need 12 liters of boiling water and 1 to 2 teaspoons of salt. What to do: Combine the salt and the boiling water.

Use this solution to thoroughly rinse your eyes.

How Often Should You Use This? You can use this mild solution to wash your eyes several times per day.

8. Vitamin supplements Your body may become deficient in vital vitamins and minerals as a result of your fast-paced lifestyle. In turn, this can make you more likely to get eye infections. Vitamins A, C, and E have been shown in studies to help maintain good health.

These nutrients may aid in the prevention of eye infections and damage. You can eat foods that are full of these nutrients. You can also eat seafood, nuts, citrus fruits, leafy vegetables, cheese, and citrus fruits.

Note: After consulting with your physician or other healthcare providers, please ensure that you take supplements.

9. Castor Oil The anti-inflammatory ricinoleic acid found in castor oil was found to reduce eye swelling in animal studies (9). Additionally, the oil may

lubricate your eyes, which may alleviate any irritation.

Castor oil (100 percent organic, cold-pressed, and free of hexane) Sterile washcloth Water What to Do: Apply castor oil to your eyes.

After the washcloth has been soaked in warm water, place it over your eyes. Ten minutes is about right.

How Often Should You Perform This? Perform this twice daily.

Related: The Ten Best Uses, Health Benefits, and Negative Effects of Castor Oil Cold

Compress Putting an eye infection's inflammation and discomfort under a cold compress can help reduce them. However, the infection will not be treated by it.

What to Do: Apply a cold compress to the affected eye for about two to three minutes. You will need one.

Repeat this twice more.

How Often Should You Perform This? Perform this procedure two times per day until the swelling goes down.

You may be able to effectively manage the infection with the assistance of these home remedies. However, it is always preferable to avoid infection altogether.

Several preventative measures are available to you:

Do not rub your eyes or contact them with unclean hands.   Makeup, towels, and handkerchiefs should not be shared with others.

Avoid wearing contacts at night.

Make sure your contact lenses are clean and changed every three months.

Eliminate your eye makeup before bed..

Keep your spectacles to yourself.

Protect your eyes from pollution and dust as you dry.

How to Get Better Eyesight
Ten Ways to Improve Your Vision Getting regular eye exams is one way to improve your vision and avoid injuries or illnesses that could hurt it. Read on to learn more about other ways to improve your vision.

1. Make sure you get enough of the essential vitamins and minerals Vitamins A, C, and E, in addition to the mineral zinc, contain antioxidants that can help stop macular degeneration. The macula, the part of the eye that controls central vision, deteriorates in this condition.

These vital nutrients can be found in a wide range of colorful fruits and vegetables, such as:
carrots, red peppers, broccoli, spinach, strawberries, sweet potatoes, and citrus fruits are all good sources of omega-3 fatty acids, and salmon and flaxseed are two of the best.

2. Carotenoids and a few other nutrients are also important for improving vision. Carotenoids like lutein and zeaxanthin, which are found in the retina, are two examples. They can also be found in leafy green foods, eggs, broccoli, and zucchini.
Supplements containing lutein and zeaxanthin are also an option. By absorbing blue and ultraviolet light and increasing the macula's pigment density, these carotenoids protect the eye.

3. Maintain your fitness Yes, working out and eating well can benefit your eyes as well as your waistline. Eye blood vessels can be damaged by type 2 diabetes, which is more common in people who are overweight or obese.

Trusted Source, this condition is known as diabetic retinopathy. Your arteries' delicate walls are damaged when you have too much sugar in your blood. Your retina, the back of your eye that is sensitive to light, has very small arteries that leak blood and fluid into the eye, affecting your vision.

Your risk of developing type 2 diabetes and its numerous complications can be reduced by regularly checking your blood sugar levels and remaining fit and trim.

4. Manage long-term conditions Diabetes isn't the only illness that can affect your vision. Your eyesight may also be affected by other conditions, such as multiple sclerosis and high blood pressure, according to Trusted Source. Chronic inflammation, which can harm your health from head to toe, is linked to these conditions.

As an illustration, irritation of the optic nerve can result in pain and, surprise, total vision loss. You can't prevent a disease like multiple sclerosis, but you can try to control it with healthy habits and medication.

Antihypertensive medications, a heart-healthy diet, and exercise are all effective treatments for high blood pressure.

5. Protect your eyes with appropriate eyewear whether you're playing racquetball, working in your garage, or participating in a school science experiment.

If there is a possibility that chemicals, sharp objects, or materials like wood shavings, metal shards, or even a stray elbow during a basketball game could get into your eye, tough, protective eyewear is necessary.

Trusted Source uses a polycarbonate that is about ten times stronger than other plastics to make a lot of protective goggles.

Look for safety goggles.

6. Sunglasses aren't just for looking cool, either. One of the most important things you can do to improve your vision is to wear shades. Sunglasses that

completely shield you from the sun's UVA and UVB rays should be your top choice.

Sunglasses protect your eyes from conditions caused by damage to the eyes. These include apterygial, a tissue growth over the white part of the eye, cataracts, and macular degeneration. Tergum's can cause astigmatism, which can blur the vision Trusted Source.

Additionally, wearing a hat with a wide brim can protect your eyes from sun damage.

7. Follow the rule of 20-20-20. Your eyes work hard during the day and require periodic breaks. If you spend a lot of time working at a computer, the strain can be especially severe. Follow the 20-20-20 rule to reduce stress Trusted Source

That means you should look at something 20 feet away for 20 seconds every 20 minutes instead of at your computer.

8. Stop smoking. You know that smoking harms your lungs, heart, teeth, skin, and just about every other part of your body. That also applies to your eyes. Your risk of developing cataracts and age-

related macular degeneration is significantly increased if you smoke.

Fortunately, within the first few hours of quitting, your eyes, lungs, heart, and other body parts can begin to recover from years of damage caused by tobacco. Additionally, your blood vessels will benefit more and inflammation will lessen throughout your eyes and the rest of your body the longer you refrain from smoking.

9. Learn about your family's eye health history Some eye conditions are passed down from generation to generation. Knowing about eye conditions that your parents or grandparents had can help you take preventative measures.

Conditions inherited include:

age-related macular degeneration optic atrophy glaucoma retinal degeneration
10. Knowing your family's history can help you take early precautions. Keep your hands and lenses clean because your eyes are particularly susceptible to infections and germs. Your vision can be affected by even simple eye irritations. Because of these factors,

you should always wash your hands after handling your contact lenses or touching your eyes.

In addition, it's critical that you follow the directions and wash your hands and disinfect your contact lenses Trusted Source.

Your doctor or the manufacturer of your contact lenses should also tell you when to change them. Eye bacterial infections can result from germs in your contact lenses.

Natural remedies that might be effective for hazy vision

Natural treatments for blurry vision Depending on the cause, these natural treatments and changes to your lifestyle may help you see more clearly:

1. Rest and recuperation Human eyes are delicate and require rest just like the rest of your body; consequently, ensure that you get adequate sleep. Using the 20-20-20 rule, take breaks every 20 minutes if you spend a lot of time at a computer.

Simply shift your focus to something at least 20 feet away for 20 seconds every 20 minutes to follow the 20-20-20 rule.

2. Lubricate the eyes If dry eyes are the cause of your blurry vision, blinking a few times or gently massaging the eyelids with a warm compress may help. The meibomian, or oil, glands in the eyelid may be triggered by this.

Artificial tears can also be purchased over the counter at a local pharmacy or online. These prevent strain-induced dry eyes by keeping the eyes lubricated.

If you live in a dry area, use a humidifier to improve the quality of the air. Particularly at night, try to avoid having air blow directly at your face.

3. Stop smoking. Smoking can cause many eye diseases, such as amyotrophic lateral sclerosis, cataracts, and damage to the optic nerve. Additionally, smoking cigarettes can aggravate dry eyes.

4. Avoiding allergens is the first step in treating and preventing allergies.

For instance, if you are allergic to dust, you should make it a habit to clean your bedroom on a regular basis to keep dust from building up and getting in your eyes while you sleep.

Close the windows and utilize an allergen-filtering air conditioner if your allergies are caused by the outdoors.
You can also ask your doctor about antihistamine eye drops if these methods don't work. Some are available without a prescription, while others can be purchased over the counter (OTC).

5. Take omega-3 fatty acids. Research shows that people with dry eye symptoms can benefit from omega-3 fatty acids. Additional study is required to verify these results, though. You can get omega-3 fatty acids from supplements, but you can also get them from eating more of the following:
omega-3 supplements should be discussed with a medical professional before taking them. This is because they might make bleeding more likely.

Wearing sunglasses when outside in the sun is one way to protect your eyes. Select sunglasses that are resistant to both UVA and UVB rays.
In dry, cold weather or when snow on the ground reflects the sun into your eyes, sunglasses can also be useful. They prevent the wind from irritating the eyes, which is another advantage.

6. Taking vitamin A

A diet devoid of vitamin A-rich foods can cause dry eyes and other vision issues, such as blurry vision.

There are two types of vitamin A:

protamine and carotenoids, which are found in plant-based foods like retinol and retinyl esters, which are found in animal products like dairy, liver, and fish

Sweet potatoes, carrots, kale, red peppers, spinach, and butternut squash are all sources of protamine A carotenoids, which, according to studies conducted by Trusted Source, may significantly lower the risk of AMD. Keep in mind that for men and women, the recommended daily allowance (RDA) for vitamin A is 900 micrograms (mcg) and 700 mcg, respectively.

While taking a vitamin A supplement may lower your risk of developing AMD and other eye conditions, exercise caution.

Vitamin A dissolves in fat. As a result, it is stored in your body and has the potential to build up to unhealthy levels over time. Vitamin A overdose can cause toxicity and serious side effects.

Make sure to properly clean your contact lenses and wash your hands if you wear them if you do. If you follow the provided instructions, contact lenses can be disinfected. Avoid wearing your contact lenses to bed because doing so can be risky.

Chapter 5

Ways to Avoid Blindness and Preserve Your Vision

If you've never had a vision problem, you probably don't think much about your eyes. Additionally, you may not be aware of the changes that come with age, some of which can have a significant impact on your vision or even result in blindness.

The good news is that even simple preventative measures like wearing sunglasses and eating greens can help preserve your vision and prevent vision issues in later life.

The following is a list of ten eye facts that will assist you in preserving your vision and eye health for many years to come.

1. Your eye health depends on what you eat. The No. 1 is to eat well. One way to care for your eyes, according to Rebecca Taylor, M.D., a spokesperson for the American Academy of Ophthalmology and an ophthalmologist at Nashville Vision Associates in Tennessee. Additionally, she suggests aiming to get your nutrients from food: Instead of taking vitamins, eat them.
What should the design of your eye-healthy plate be? Similar to any good, nutritious meal. Dr. Taylor starts with a big salad of spinach or kale with colorful vegetables on top. According to the AAO, green leafy vegetables contain the nutrients lutein and zeaxanthin, which have been shown to lower the risk of eye diseases. According to the National Institutes of Health, vitamin A in bright yellow and orange vegetables like carrots and sweet potatoes

improves eye health. Fruits like mangoes, strawberries, and oranges contain vitamin C and other antioxidants, which Taylor claims also aid in the fight against eye disease. She also eats salmon or other cold-water fish in her ideal diet because omega-3 fatty acids are good for making tears, which helps with dry eyes.

2. Comprehensive eye exams catch problems with a vision early. The only way to detect a wide range of issues, including glaucoma and diabetic eye disease, and to ensure that you receive prompt treatment, is to have an annual eye exam. To ensure that their vision has not changed, the majority of people with vision problems should visit their eye doctor once a year.

The AAO recommends the following schedule for the rest of us:

At 40: a basic eye exam for people aged 40 to 55: an eye exam every two to four years for people 55 to 64: an eye exam every one to three years for people over 65: an annual eye exam Your eye doctor will take a history of your family, examine your pupils, central vision, color vision, and eye pressure. Using special eye drops, he or she will also dilate or widen your pupil to see into the back of your eye and check for damage.

3. If you smoke now, you might have problems with your eyes later. Stop using any kind of tobacco, Taylor advises. Cyanide from smoke enters the bloodstream and has the potential to harm eye cells. Smoking raises your risk of developing cataracts and worsens dry eye issues. According to the Centers for Disease Control and Prevention (CDC), it also increases your risk of developing macular degeneration, which is an irreversible condition that causes vision loss in the center of the eye.

4. By shielding your eyes from the sun, you can contribute to the preservation of your vision. Taylor recommends the following eye protection: sunglasses and sunscreen. UV radiation can damage some of the driest skin on the body, including the skin around your eyes. In the eyelids and around the eyes, various types of skin cancer, including carcinoma and melanoma, can develop, causing significant damage to the eye structure.

Taylor also recommends wearing sunglasses. However, do not be deceived into thinking that darker is better. She asserts that "what matters is the sticker you peel off of the glasses when you buy them." UVA and UVB (long and short waves) rays should be completely blocked by sunglasses. The problems that lead to cataracts and macular degeneration, two common types of blindness, are sparked by ultraviolet radiation.

5. It can dry out your eyes to work all day on a computer. According to Taylor, this is in part due to the fact that we blink less when doing things near. According to American Optometric Association president Steven Loomis, OD, of Roxborough Park, Colorado, paradoxically, eye watering is one of the most common signs of dry eyes. According to him, the breakdown of the oily and mucous layers of the eyes prevents tears from evaporating, so the eye produces more water in response. Another symptom is feeling "tired eyes" at the end of the day.

Dry eyes can also result from:
Medications that cause inflammation, such as antidepressants, hormonal changes brought on by aging, and inflammation The Mayo Clinic advises looking at something at least 20 feet away every 20 minutes for 20 seconds. Dr. Loomis suggests a

warm compress and artificial tears, but not those that "get the red out" because they can prevent blood from reaching the tear glands. Restasis, a cyclosporine medication, may be prescribed by your doctor to reduce inflammation if these treatments fail.

6. In America, diabetes is the leading cause of blindness. Preventing diabetes, if at all possible, is the most effective strategy for avoiding diabetic retinopathy, the leading cause of blindness in the United States. This eye condition affects about 60% of people with type 2 diabetes and nearly all people with type 1 diabetes.

7. Macular degeneration is the leading cause of blindness after the age of 60. Macular degeneration occurs when the central part of the eye's tissue deteriorates, resulting in blurry vision or loss of vision. Macular degeneration can occur in two ways: dry and wet. In the event that fluid in the retina is the cause of vision loss, injections into the eye can be used to treat the condition. However, the majority of forms are dry and do not require treatment.
A family history of the condition, smoking (which damages the blood vessels in the eye), a diet

deficient in lutein and amaranthine, and not wearing sunglasses are all risk factors for macular degeneration.

8. Although cataract treatment is very effective, it is common. Cataracts typically begin to appear around the age of 60, making them a fairly normal part of aging. Blurred vision, faded colors, glare, diminished night vision, and double vision are all possible signs. UV rays or radiation therapy, such as cancer treatment, are linked to cataracts. According to Loomis, taking certain medications like prednisone can also make cataracts more likely. However, he adds, cataract treatment, which typically entails replacing the damaged eye lenses with new ones, is highly effective.

9. Glaucoma is caused by damage to the optic nerve in the eye. According to Loomis, this common eye condition is known for being silent and subtle. He frequently informs patients that loss of vision is the initial sign of glaucoma. According to the National Institutes of Health (NIH), an eye exam is the only method by which glaucoma can be detected and treated on its own.

When pressure builds up in the eye and starts to damage the optic nerve, glaucoma occurs.

According to Loomis, the condition progresses very slowly, and the nerve damage may take years to become severe enough to cause vision issues.

According to Loomis, diabetics and those with a family history of glaucoma are more likely to develop the condition. A once-daily eye drop that reduces eye pressure is part of most patients' treatment. Surgery might be an option if the drops don't work.

10. Your health can be seen through your eyes. According to Taylor, a person's eyes can also serve as an indicator of their overall health, despite the adage that they are the windows to their soul. In the event that a patient comes into her office with dry eyes, she asks other well-being inquiries, since having dry eyes can be a marker of rheumatoid joint pain, lupus, or thyroid sickness. Diabetes, a tumor, or a stroke could be the causes of blurry vision in patients. It's possible that people who have itchy, red eyes don't know they have an allergy to contact lenses. A patient who had unusual eye movements was also recently diagnosed with multiple sclerosis by Taylor.

Best vitamins and their foods for healthy eyes

Vitamins A, C, and E are necessary for healthy eyes. In addition, B vitamins and other nutrients may play a significant role.

Vitamin shortages may make several eye problems worse, such as glaucoma, cataracts, and age-related macular degeneration. Research suggests that several vitamin and mineral supplements could help prevent or delay the onset of these illnesses. This section focuses more on the vitamins and minerals that people need to keep their eyes healthy and how they can get them from food.

Vitamin A and vitamin A-rich food for clear vision is a component of the protein rhodopsin, which gives the eye the ability to see in low light. According to the American Academy of Ophthalmology, a deficit can cause night blindness.

Vitamin A also aids in the protection of the cornea, the eye's outermost layer. Vitamin A deficiency may cause eyes to produce insufficient moisture to maintain lubrication.

Vitamin A in humans comes primarily from beta-carotene. A carotenoid, or type of plant pigment, beta carotene can be found in a wide variety of vibrant fruits and vegetables. When carotenoids are ingested, the body turns them into vitamin A. dietary sources of vitamin A The following foods can be consumed by vitamin A-deficient individuals:

Vitamin E and foods rich in vitamin E include sweet potatoes, carrots, red peppers, pumpkin, and squash. Alpha-tocopherol is a form of vitamin E with particularly potent antioxidant properties.

Free radicals, which cause tissue damage throughout the body, are combated by antioxidants. Free radicals can occasionally harm eye proteins. Cataracts, or cloudy areas on the eye's lens, can develop as a result of this damage.

A meta-analysis conducted in 2015 came to the conclusion that taking vitamin E supplements or eating a lot of them can help lower the risk of developing cataracts.

Vitamin E-rich foods include the following:

Almonds, sunflower seeds, peanuts, safflower oil, soybean, corn, and wheat germ oil asparagus Vitamin C, and foods rich in vitamin C protect the eye from damage caused by ultraviolet light. Diet and vitamin C supplements can counteract the age-related decrease in vitamin C concentration in the eyes.

Additionally, vitamin C aids in preventing oxidative damage. Oxidative damage is a major contributor to two of the most common age-related cataracts. a reputable source for cataracts in the brain and nucleus. Nuclear cataracts occur deep within the center of the lens, whereas cortical cataracts develop on the lens's edges.

In a ten-year longitudinal study, many factors that might help in preventing the onset of nuclear cataracts were examined. There were over 1,000 pairs of female twins in the study. Participants who consumed more vitamin C had a 33% lower risk of cataract progression at the study's conclusion. Additionally, they had overall clearer lenses.

However, a review published in 2020 by Trusted Source concluded that additional research is required to fully identify the role of vitamin C as an anticataract therapy.

People are likely to have lower blood B12 levels, according to a Trusted Source review from 2015 on the topic. However, researchers found that there wasn't enough proof to draw a connection.

In this particular study, however, only women were enrolled. To support the use of B vitamins to prevent

AMD in both men and women, more study is therefore needed.

A Trusted Source study that was conducted across the country in South Korea in 2018 found a connection between glaucoma and reduced consumption of vitamin B3 (niacin). In glaucoma patients, an accumulation of fluid in the eye puts the optic nerve under pressure. As a result, vision loss may eventually result from nerve injury.

Additionally, a small 2020 study found that taking mecobalamin and vitamin B1 supplements may alleviate dry eye disease symptoms.

Foods high in B vitamins The following foods are high in B vitamins:

Foods high in B vitamins The following foods are high in B vitamins:

Vitamin B1 (thiamine): beans, lentils, pork, fish, green peas, yogurt; Vitamin B2 (riboflavin): beef, oats, yogurt, milk, clams, mushrooms, almonds; Vitamin B3 (niacin): beef liver, chicken, salmon, tuna, brown and white rice, peanuts; Vitamin B6 (pyridoxine): chickpeas; dark leafy greens; poultry; beef liver; salmon; tuna

Other nutrients for eye health

Zeaxanthin and lutein Zeaxanthin and lutein are carotenoids that are abundant in green leafy vegetables. Additionally, they are found in the eye's lens and retina.

Lutein and zeaxanthin may reduce oxidative damage to the retina as antioxidants. According to research conducted in 2017 by Trusted Source, taking approximately 6 milligrams (mg) of lutein and zeaxanthin per day may lower an individual's risk of developing AMD. Additionally, a daily dose of 0.5–1 mg may reduce the risk of glaucoma.

The following are sources of lutein and zeaxanthin:
Corn, asparagus, broccoli, lettuce, peas, kale, spinach, and spinach contain zinc. Zinc is a mineral that supports the retina, cell membranes, and protein structure of the eye.

Vitamin A can travel from the liver to the retina to produce melanin thanks to zinc. Melanin is a pigment that blocks UV light from reaching the eyes.

People who have AMD or are at risk of developing it may benefit from taking zinc supplements. The American Optometric Association says that taking certain antioxidants and 40–80 mg of zinc every day could slow the progression of advanced AMD by

25%. Additionally, it may decrease visual acuity loss by 19%.

Zinc can be obtained from:
Omega-3 fatty acids from seafood like oysters, crab, lobster turkey beans, chickpeas, nuts, pumpkin seeds, whole grains, and fortified cereals Omega-3 fatty acids from the retina of the eye The retina is shielded from degeneration and damage by these fatty acids. Omega-3 supplements have been shown to slow down age-related retinal degeneration in small animal studies. However, additional human studies are required to fully evaluate the connection.

For the treatment of dry eye syndrome, many doctors suggest using omega-3 fatty acids from a trusted source. A person who suffers from dry eye syndrome is unable to produce sufficient tears to maintain eye lubrication. However, a large randomized control trial found that placebo did not significantly alleviate dry eye symptoms.

The following are foods high in omega-3 fatty acids: Oily fish like sardines, tuna, and herring, as well as flaxseed, walnuts, and chia seeds. Vitamins and a healthy diet for healthy eyes A healthy, well-balanced diet can help protect a person's vision and promote good eye health. Frequently, a varied diet with a number of nutrient-dense foods can supply an adequate amount of each vitamin and mineral. However, if a person's diet does not meet their nutritional needs, they may need to take additional supplements to meet certain goals.

Supplements can sometimes cause side effects, so it's important to talk to your doctor before making big changes to your diet. Chapter 6 Nutrient-rich foods to improve eye health In this section, we examine the evidence for ten nutrient-rich foods to improve eye health. For instance, taking large amounts of zinc can affect how the body absorbs it. We also talk about eye health warning signs and other ways to keep your eyes healthy.

Chapter 6

Foods high in nutrients to improve eye health

The American Optometric Association (AOA) and the American Academy of Ophthalmology (AAO) continue to recommend the top 10 foods for eye health based on the AREDS studies.

According to AREDS data, the following 10 foods are particularly rich in nutrients:

1. A healthy lifestyle can help reduce the likelihood of acquiring eye diseases.

Several fish have large amounts of omega-3 fatty acids.

Oily fish have oil in their guts and body tissues, hence they have a higher concentration of omega-3-rich fish oil than other fish. The fish that contain the most of the advantageous omega-3 fatty acids are the ones listed below:

Fish oil can be found in tuna, salmon, trout, mackerel, sardines, anchovies, and herring, among other foods. According to some research, fish oil can be used to cure dry eyes, including those brought on by prolonged computer use.

2. Omega-3 fatty acids are also abundant in nuts and legumes. Additionally, nuts contain a lot of vitamin E, which can help protect the eyes from damage caused by aging.

Nuts can be purchased online and in most grocery stores following seeds, legumes, and nuts are good for the eyes.. cashews, peanuts, Brazil nuts, lentils, and walnuts SeedS, Like Nuts and legumes, are a good source of vitamins E and high in omega-3 fatty acids. You can buy seeds in most grocery stores and online. Omega-3-rich seeds include:

hemp seeds, flax seeds, and chia seeds Citrus fruits contain a lot of vitamin C, which, like vitamin E, is an antioxidant that the AOA recommends for preventing age-related damage to the eyes.

Citrus fruits high in vitamin C include:
grapefruits, oranges, and lemons Vegetables with leafy greens are a good source of vitamin C, which is good for the eyes, and they are also high in lutein and zeaxanthin.

spinach, kale, and collards Carrots Carrots contain a lot of beta carotene and Vitamin A. Carrots acquire their orange color from beta carotene.

Vitamin A from a trusted source is necessary for clear vision. It is a component of rhodopsin, a protein that aids the retina in absorbing light.

Although the body needs beta-carotene to make vitamin A, research on its role in vision is mixed. Sweet potatoes contain a lot of beta-carotene as carrots do. Additionally, they are a good source of the antioxidant vitamin E. Beef Zinc, which has been linked to improved long-term eye health, is abundant in beef. Zinc can help prevent macular degeneration and age-related sight loss.

Zinc is abundant in the eye itself, particularly in the retina and the vascular tissue that surrounds it.

Zinc can also be found in pork loin and chicken breast, albeit in lower amounts than beef.

9. Lutein and amaranthine, which can lower the risk of age-related sight loss, can be found in abundance in eggs. Eggs are also a good source of zinc and vitamins C and E.

10. Water is a fluid that is necessary for life and also essential for eye health.
Dehydration can be avoided by drinking a lot of water, which may help alleviate dry eye symptoms.

Drinks and foods that harm the eyes The same healthy diet that is good for your heart is good for your eyes. Your eyes and your heart are both vascular, which means they contain blood vessels.
The retina, the light-sensitive tissue at the back of the eye, receives oxygen and nutrients from the tiny blood vessels known as capillaries in the eyes. Plaque or fatty deposits from unhealthy foods can quickly clog these small vessels.
The majority of us are generally aware that processed foods are harmful. Your vision and heart health are both affected by this. The following foods are bad for your eyes:

1: White foods like white pasta, bread, and rice are made up of simple carbohydrates. They raise blood sugar because they are quickly digested and absorbed. Hyperglycemia, or high blood sugar, has been linked to cataracts, age-related macular degeneration, and diabetic retinopathy.

Additionally, eating a diet high in simple carbohydrates can lead to weight gain and raise your risk of heart disease and high cholesterol. Additionally, despite the fact that you may find that they are delectable and that they make you want more, they do not provide any real nutritional value. All of the nutrients, vitamins, and fiber in these foods are removed because they have either been bleached or processed.

2: High-Sodium Foods Consuming a diet high in sodium can cause hypertension or high blood pressure. High sodium levels are linked to cataract development, according to research.
The blood vessels in the retina that are affected by hypertension can also be damaged. The retina suffers vascular injury as a result of hypertension. It can affect vision if not treated and diagnosed promptly.

Sodium-rich foods include:
3: Pickles, hot dogs, bacon, deli meats, and canned goods Saturated and trans fats are unhealthy fats that can cause plaque buildup in vessels and raise blood cholesterol levels. Additionally, these fats may prevent the eyes from absorbing certain nutrients

that are essential to their health and protection against eye diseases.

Saturated and trans-fat-rich foods include:
4: Margarine, French fries, cookies, potato chips, meat, and dairy products Toppings, dressings, and condiments Your refrigerator door probably contains condiments, dressings, and toppings. The following are fattening options:

Mayonnaise
Salad dressings
Jam
5: Drinks with added sugar include energy drinks, sports drinks, and soda. Diabetes, heart disease, and eye diseases are more likely to occur in people with high sugar intake.
 Advice for Preventing Dry Eyes Everyone at Grin Eye Care is anticipating spring because of Kansas City's rising temperatures, although it still feels like winter most of the time. One of the most typical issues during the chilly winter months is dryness.

Check out these five strategies to prevent dry eyes and maintain the happiness and health of your eyes.

1 ADD HEAT TO YOUR HOME: Use a humidifier to rehydrate the dry air in your home.

2. Select the appropriate eye drops: A great way to keep your eyes lubricated is to use artificial tears three to four times a day. Systane, Refresh, Soothe, and Blink is excellent choices. Avoid drops that claim to alleviate redness, like Visine, because they are more irritating. We are happy to answer any questions you may have over the phone and can recommend the best eye drop for you.

3. RECEIVE A BREAK: Make sure you take frequent breaks from staring at the screen if you are one of the millions of people who spend their day working at a computer. A major cause of dry eyes is a strain on the digital eye. Follow the rule of 20-20-20: Every 20 minutes, look 20 feet for at least 20 seconds without looking at your screen. For more details, see our blog post about Digital Eye Strain.

4. ADD MORE OMEGA-3 FATTY ACIDS TO YOUR DIET: Omega-3 fatty acids improve the health of the oil glands at the base of the eyelashes and the quality of the tear film. Omega-3s are

abundant in fish oil supplements and foods like salmon, eggs, spinach, walnuts, and soybeans. Make sure to inquire about the best brands of supplements from our reputable eye doctors if you intend to take them.

5. GET YOUR MAKEUP CLEANED UP: To prevent the growth of bacteria, wash your makeup brushes and replace your eye makeup, particularly mascara. The oil glands can become clogged with bacteria, which can cause dryness. Skin creams containing retinol—another cause of dry eyes—may also be something you should steer clear of. Every night, before going to bed, remove your makeup. Coconut oil is an excellent natural alternative to store-bought makeup removers.

6. APPLY ARMORED COMPRESSES: One of the best ways to open up the oil glands and keep your tear film healthy is to apply a warm beaded eye mask or washcloth to your eyes for five minutes. To prevent the tears from evaporating too quickly, the glands at the base of the eyelashes secrete an oil layer into the tear film. Clean the lashes and lids with baby shampoo or lid scrubs after applying the warm compress. To keep the eyes moist, a healthy tear film is necessary.

7. CONSERVE YOUR EYES: Wear 100% UV-protective sunglasses to shield your eyes from the wind and cold air if you are going to be outside in the cold weather. We have a great selection of frames, including the most popular brands, in our optical shop. When you are driving, you should also keep the heat vents away from your face because the hot air can quickly dry out your eyes, causing excessive watering, dryness, and discomfort.

8. Reduce your time spent in contact: Overwearing contact lenses are known to worsen dry eyes. During these dry winter months, give your eyes a break and wear your glasses more often. Always replace your contact lenses in accordance with your eye doctor's recommendations and avoid sleeping with them on.

9. Schedule a consultation with one of our doctors: Our trusted doctors are here to examine, treat, and manage all levels and types of dry eye, which can be caused by a variety of factors. Over 4 million people, according to the National Institutes of Health, suffer from dry eye disease. Dry eye disease is a medical condition that can be treated in a variety of ways. If you're one of the millions of people who

suffer from dry eye, give us a call right away to schedule an appointment and get some relief.

10. Consume water: One of the best and easiest ways to keep your skin and eyes moisturized is to drink enough water. Try to consume eight glasses of 8 ounces each day.

Healthy eating equals healthy vision The expression "you are what you eat" is spot-on. Heart health and overall health are linked to eye health.
By replacing foods that are bad for your eyes with foods that are good for your heart and eyes, you can keep a healthy diet. This can help you avoid certain eye conditions and lower your risk of getting them.

Los Angeles Eye Care is the place to go if you have questions or concerns about your eye health

Conclusions

Damage brought on by aging affects more than only the eyes. Age-related changes in the eyes can include things like eyelid thinning and difficulties concentrating on close objects, although they are not life-threatening. Some alterations, though, can cause major eye problems that could endanger your vision. As we age, the eyes start to lose their capacity to stay moisturized. As a result, eyes may become inflamed, sticky, dry, or gritty. The lens of the eye may become less elastic over time. Moreover, night vision may start to worsen, creating difficulties for nighttime driving. On the other hand, macular degeneration, cataracts, and diabetes retinopathy can cause blindness.

How can you determine whether an eye condition is merely bothersome or the start of something more serious? If you suffer any of the following symptoms, contact your doctor right once. Early identification of major eye diseases can help you preserve your vision. You can take care of eye disorders that do not endanger your eyesight in order to maintain your eyes pleasant and your vision as clear as feasible.